"It is towards the future that we have labored with these concepts, to make them understandable, workable and tremendously effective. We hope others will seize this work and blaze a new pathway that does not use the old and outdated management approaches"
—Paul Snyder

I0480245

MANAGING IN PHARMACEUTICAL SALES... PEARLS AMONG THE OCEANS OF STRATEGIES

<u>WHAT</u> YOU REALLY NEED TO MANAGE

WITH SPECIAL EMPHASIS ON:

- The dreaded recruiting & hiring process
- Planning: 80% thinking; 20% writing; 100% doing
- How To Open all channels of communication
- No fluff ideas on building a team
- Coaching & Counseling…Our Thoughts
- A practical method to making decisions

SHEELEY CONSULTING GROUP, LLC

Consulting: Sales: Marketing: Advertising:Management: Publications

Published by:

A Book's Mind

PO Box 272847

Fort Collins, CO 80527

ACKNOWLEDGMENTS

Paul and I are grateful to the many friends of distinction who have contributed to the content and writing of this book and the other two books we have written. In particular, special thanks to my daughter Stacy who helped us find Brian Dunne the best website design guy on this planet, and for all her ideas on layout design and content. I would also like to give thanks to Dave Beckwith, Mike Monti , Ann Grana, Peter Bornstein and Henry Trenkle for their insightful comments, suggestions, and editing work. To Charley McLeskey, MD, Astra Zeneca, for his years of friendship and for his ideas on what title to give each book. Thank you to my wife, Diane, for her sage advice with this book. In addition, to Floyd Orfield and his team at *"A Book's Mind"* for cover design and publishing. They are the best in the business. These books could not have been written alone by either Paul or me…it was the synergy between us that captured all of these concepts and made them understandable. As Paul said, *"we hope others will seize this work and blaze a new pathway that does not use the old and barren promotional approaches."* We hope you do. It was a great, once-in-a-lifetime opportunity to work with Paul in writing these three books; he is truly a genius in the pharmaceutical arena.

The years teach much which the days never know" —Ralph Waldo Emerson

FOREWORD

It was a call I received from a pharmaceutical teaching-hospital representative, who called on the University of Arizona and the University of New Mexico, that prompted the writing of this book. He had just been promoted to a District Sales Manager, and called to ask me for advice on what were the key elements to manage and <u>how to manage what was</u> <u>really important to manage</u>. The new management position he accepted was supervising office-based representatives.

Two weeks after the representative called, we were asked by a pharmaceutical company to put together a two-day management training class for their new and experienced field-based managers, we immediately thought that it was not possible to do a class on how to be a *"good"* pharmaceutical field-manager in 2-days.

What convinced us to accept the company's offer to teach a 2-day class and to provide the representative recently promoted to District Sales Manager was our interest in delving into what a manager, particularly a new manager, really needed to know to get off on the right foot.

What were the real elements of management that we needed to teach? What did they really need to know? We asked former past managers their thoughts. We spent a lot of time discussing this with current managers we knew.

It was the years of being a front-line manager faced with thousands of decisions which provided *The Rest of the Story*…here are our thoughts and observations on what we agreed were the real elements of management. In other words, based on our many years of managing and working with office-based, teaching-hospital based and Medical Science Liaison PharmD's calling on "*thought leaders*", if you can put into practice what we are providing for you to learn in this book, we feel you will be on your way to being a success as a manager.

We are particularly interested in your feedback and comments relative to the concepts and "*management maxims*" we outlined in this book, and would welcome the opportunity to consult with your management team.

Please let us know your thoughts.

Ron Sheeley   Paul Snyder
Rsheeley09@gmail.com   Psnyder1@indy.rr.com

CHAPTER ONE
INTERVIEWING AND HIRING

"When it comes to making a final hiring decision between two equally qualified candidates, the hungrydog hunts best" –Bob Suffill

THE DREADED RECRUITING AND HIRING PROCESS

Of all the management skills needed to be successful, the ability to hire the right candidate was on the top of the list in the minds of most of the experienced managers we talked with. And, what we tried to put together in this section is a list of items we felt were critical to successful hiring that what we learned and observed over the countless interviews we conducted as District Sales Managers.

Here are our thoughts on recruiting and hiring.

What is the mission? Establish a clear, concise mission statement on what is the anticipated outcome. The mission statement sets the direction, pace and outcome of the whole recruiting process. The successful result of a top notch hire is the first step in growing a more productive and dynamic sales staff. So there is a lot riding on this mission!

Common pitfalls in the recruiting and hiring process: Relying on old technology. Many major pharma companies still take an inordinate amount of time to gain a hire. This is counter-productive to the results expected from filling the opening. Suitable candidates may move on to other opportunities because of "the waiting game".

Poorly conceived want ads.

Since a clear mission statement defines outcome, be sure that the Want Ad states in clear terms just what your expectations are of the candidate. Are you looking for previous pharma sales experience or, more broadly, outside sales experience?

What other experience or special attributes are desired? When giving out information on where to send respondent resumes, be sure to build in *fire walls*.

Lack of coordination of management interview team. Often there is a lack of management motivation and commitment due to several factors. The hiring process is often seen as an additional burden apart from the day-to-day management function. When, in fact, the recruiting and hiring process is a *key* management function. This awareness yields additional stress. Let's face it. There is a lot riding on decisions that are made here. What are the best ways to address what is really a made-to-order opportunity to upgrade staff?

How proper screening sets the pace for the entire process: If your program has the ability for the candidate to respond via the intenet then you can simply download off the site and print up the resume and cover letter. What are you looking for in a resume and cover letter? The cover letter is your first insight into the candidate's ability to communicate in a clear, logical and grammatical way. What are the "red flags" and knock-out factors to look for? What are your preferences? Once you have scanned all the resumes that, hopefully, were generated by your ad, how do you get organized for the next step? Stack them with best on top and start there. We think the proper screening of resumes is critical to the success of getting the best candidate. When you receive over

1,000 resumes for a single vacant territory it is important to set up parameters of what you are looking for from the start to save time in getting to the top applicants.

How to set up a Telephone Screening Interview. Once you have winnowed the batch of resumes and graded them, start with your *"A"* clutch. At this time, before beginning the screens, you'll need to establish an interview site (see **"Fire Walls"** below). How do you determine how much time to invest in First Interviews? Create a Day Interview Scheduling Guide…We show you how as well as how to track progress. How do you decide when a successful Screen takes place? What is the next logical step that gets you and the candidate to the interview site and at the same times maintains your *fire walls?* What procedure is put into place should the situation arise where the candidate can't make the interview? This important step can save you time wasted.

How to conduct a Telephone Screening Interview. When the candidate picks up on your call introduce yourself, with your company affiliation and title. Knowing what questions to ask will save time and move the decision making process along on whether or not an interview is warranted. Have a cue sheet or form to help. What kind of information from the candidate will help you to close out the screen? What background information does this candidate have regarding this type of sales? Is there a potential match between expectations and reality? Have you confirmed with the candidate your company's requirements and their ability to meet these requirements? What are your requirements? Knowing what questions to ask as follow-up for comparison and confirmation of earlier responses is a key skill set. Now it's decision time. How do you get to the next step?

Working within management manpower resources and limitations: One face-to-face interview or a team approach? What are the advantages and disadvantages of each? For instance, a one interview only approach can compress the time needed to gain a hire. Then again, a team effort can add variety to the task.

A team spirit adds an element of drama and fun since it's a shared experience. As a former highly rated boss use to say to me, *"Hire in haste and repent at leisure."* Efficiency and speed should not be confused with haste.

Preparation for the interview: You expect the candidate to be prepared for the interview and the candidate expects the same from you! Lack of preparation by the interviewer is not only counterproductive; it's just plain bad manners! This reflects poorly not only on the recruiter but also on the company. We take you through, step-by-step, so that you are prepared and primed for the interview. We show you what areas are ripe for follow-up and "drill down" questions. Under education note in particular claims as to organizations and involvement, offices held and accomplishments. This can be an area of exaggeration or worse.   Hobbies or interests are also an area where exaggeration sometimes is discovered. An example: *"Jogger and Competitive Runner"*. What event(s) did he or she run in? Was length of race in kilometers or miles? How fast was your time? What's been your best individual effort and at what event? (Follow-up questions that can smoke out false claims.) Be careful of what you write, and where you write notes during the interview.

The interview: The cover letter, resume and telephone screening guide are the touchstones for the interview along with any other paperwork generated in the meantime. Set the tone of the interview as professional and friendly rather than confrontational and interrogatorial. Plumb applicant understanding and background knowledge of the industry, company and job. What else do you need to "check out"? For example, is eye contact appropriate? When answering questions, does the candidate gaze upward and to the left? Why is this a *red flag*?

The "Ostrich Effect" and other interview pitfalls to avoid: The *"ostrich effect"*…with head down, writing too much and not really observing candidate in action. In response to your questions ask yourself, *"What is he/she really telling me?"* Impressions: open and straight forward (positive) or indirect and manufactured for consumption (negative). The tendency of the interviewer is to become too involved in filling out the interview form rather than staying involved with the subject. We teach you how to move beyond this and remain connected with and focused on the interviewee. Another pitfall, for example, is including the answer within the question. Why is this and what can be done to avoid this "leading the witness" behavior? When are follow-up and drill down questions called for?

Fire Walls and building security safeguards: In this day and age we as managers and recruiter/interviewers need to design in safeguards that protect us through the entire R & H process. Why? If the candidate is not satisfied with your follow-up or lack thereof...you have a potentially angry and possibly obsessive individual who may pester you with callbacks or worse. What can you do to avoid this? We show you! Where possible the location should be in a public place. What you are obviously protecting yourself against is a salacious allegation from an unhappy or unbalanced interviewee. But what kind of public place? We tell you. What kind of arrangements need to be made before the interview? Our experience here can assure a smooth running interview process.

SOME SAMPLE QUESTIONS FOR THE INTERVIEW:

- *"What brings you here today?"*

- *"Tell me about your most recent employment."*

- *"Under what situations or conditions do you perform at your best?"*

- *"What have you done recently in the area of self-improvement?"*

- *"Tell me about a decision you made or action you took that you later regretted."*

- *"What do you do for exercise"?*

- *"At this point in the interview what would you like to know more about?"*

- *"What's the most important attribute or attributes to making an effective sales presentation?"*

- *"Why should we hire you?!"*

This is just a sampling of the many questions you have to select from to customize each interview to each candidate.

Response and Follow-Up: Let's take a closer look at Response and Follow-Up Questions as a skill set. For the purpose of illustration we'll select the Response Question…"*What prompted your move from company B to company A?*" At this point you have no idea in which direction this query will take you. In a way you have passed control of the interview to the interviewee.

The response might be… *"I saw it as an opportunity to grow my career."* Here your Follow-Up Question might be *"How so?"* (Simple and Non-directive) What is happening is that now the candidate must explain himself (herself) with some convincing specifics.

Each response from the candidate generates your next Follow-Up Question. We teach you this skill. This skill set takes on the feeling and excitement of a chess match!

The more often you apply the technique the more skillful you become and the more fun you'll experience with the whole *"Dreaded Recruiting & Hiring Process"*.

Decision time: The importance of that *"gut feeling"*…Good, bad or indifferent? Your gut feelings are based on your previous experiences…don't discount them. Instead try to identify and define the basis for that feeling. Certainly, we want as interviewers to be fair, legally and politically correct and objective. However, as managers, we are expected to make decisions and to some degree subjectivity must play a role…nothing wrong with that. What is important? Consistency, Constancy and Integrity.

The Applicant: Up till now neither business etiquette nor legal concerns require you or your company to correspond with any candidates following terminal interviews. Should you determine at the end of a first interview that the candidate does not make the cut? What do you say to end the process? When you decide to move on to a second interview with the candidate's agreement, this is when the Application is usually tendered. The other option, if using an onsite team approach is to tender the Application following a successful Second Interview. When the Application is received back from the Applicant your obligations have increased both legally and professionally. We show you how to avoid the *"mine fields"*. In some happy situations you may find you have more qualified Applicants than you do openings. What do you do if this occurs?

The Application: Most companies have in place support services to assist the manager in checking out facts as stated in writing by the Applicant. If the driving record indicates more than one moving violation within the last three years…this is usually a knockout factor (Covered with the candidate during the Telephone Screen.). If the Applicant is asked to give employment, business and personal references, these are checked out via telephone inquiries. The Application is treated as a legal declaration and document from the Applicant. How do you verify a college degree? There's an easy way. Any falsification is cause for disqualification. When all checks out to the hiring manager's satisfaction, then a call can be put through to the Applicant with the job offer. What do you need to do as a matter of record? If the Applicant accepts, what do you need to do to complete the hire? Then it's *"high fives"!* You have completed your mission.

INTERVIEWING AND HIRING

In this section we will explore interview questions we have asked applicants with previous pharmaceutical sales experience and candidates with no previous pharmaceutical sales experience that we feel accomplish two things:

- Provide the person being interviewed with an opportunity to express their comments on questions which get to the core of pharmaceutical sales.

- Provide the manager with an opportunity to analyze and weigh carefully candidate responses.

Further, we will provide insight into what to listen/look for in candidate responses to each question. The what to **"Look For"** following each interview question provides insight into what we think the interviewer should question relative to the candidate's response. For new managers, the what to **"Look For"** questions are invaluable.

PART I: PREVIOUS PHARMACEUTICAL SALES EXPERIENCE

Does candidate talk in terms of establishing projects and contacting key physicians?

Does the candidate talk about establishing a promotional spend budget for each product?

"Tell me about your experiences in promoting products to (name of physician specialty)

Look For

- Determining who the top prescribers are in the territory.
- Importance of developing rapport and trust.

"Describe your last work week, day-by-day, in segments of time"?

Look For

- Why did they set up their schedule that way?
- How did the schedule work?
- Could the schedule been improved? How?

- Did they quit at 3pm?

- Did they attend any evening business activities?

"What will you approach be at a first display in a physician's office?

Look For

- What they plan to use (clinical study, file card, literature, etc.) to sell physician?

- Does candidate talk about probing physician to find out types of patients the physician sees?

- Does the candidate talk about developing rapport with the office manager? Office staff?

A physician in your territory has closed access to Reps. How do you proceed?

Look For

- Seeing the physician outside the office, e.g., hospital, hospice or nursing home.

- Seeking help from a 'friendly' physician to assist in seeing physician.

- Talking to the office RN.

"Describe how you would set up a project to sell a product that was minimally selling?"

Look For

- Investigating which competitive product(s) are selling.

- Gather info/studies/package inserts to compete against competition.

- Define the key physician targets.

"You have 3-drugs to promote to different physician specialties. How do you decide: What to do? Where to go? How to budget your promotional funds?

Look For

- Does the candidate talk about spending time selling the drug with the best return on invested time?

- Does the candidate talk about the challenges?

"How do you offset the competition? What challenges did you find"?

Look For

- How the candidate compared his product(s) to the competition, i.e., did they build on their product or tear down the competitor's product?

- What did they use to combat the competition?

- Good to ask for specific examples here.

List the products you promoted. How did each do at the end of the year?

Look For

- How many drugs they promoted last year?

- Which drugs did better than others? Ask specific questions why some drugs did better than others.

How do you use clinical reprints?

Look For

- How do they talk about using reprints in a sales situation? Do they consider reprints important?

- Does the candidate talk about how they break down a reprint to present it during a sales presentation?

PART II---NO PHARMACEUTICAL SALES EXPERIENCE

What brings you here today?

Look for

- Does the candidate talk about looking for a job or a career?

- Does the candidate talk about specific reasons he wants a career in pharmaceutical sales?

Tell me about your most recent employment

Look for

- Does the candidate discuss past successful sales experience?

- Does candidate bad-mouth present or former employer?

- What they learned on former jobs?

Under what situations or conditions do you perform at your best?

Look for

- What does the candidate say about stressful situations or 'time crunches'?

- How does candidate handle rejection?

- What was your most difficult college class? Why?

What do you do for exercise?

Look for

- While not a knock-out question, it takes a lot of energy to do the job of the pharmaceutical sales Rep…up/down and in-out all day.

- Is the candidate a coach-potato?

What have you done in the area of self-development?

Look for

- Look for specific examples here.

Tell me about a decision or action you took that you later regretted?

Look for

- Specific examples.

- Was action or decision career oriented?

- How did you follow up afterwards?

What is the most important attribute or attributes to making an effective sales Presentation?

Look for

- Does candidate talk about persistence?

- Does candidate discuss importance of knowing one's product?

- Does candidate mention sales skills? If so, which skill?

Why should we hire you?

Look for

- Does candidate talk about ability to go the extra mile?

- Ability and desire to learn?

- Is he/she a Team player?

CHAPTER TWO
REPRESENTATIVE TRIP REPORTS

The report you write following a working trip with a representative in the field, aka the *Representative Trip Report* (RTR), in our opinion, is not only the sole document you have to record the actual activities and sales skills the sales representative displays while working in the field, but is an important part of the entire counseling, evaluation and appraisal process. The trip report allows you, the manager, the opportunity to:

- Praise Representative performance – always start with a positive.

- Document areas in which the representative needs improvement.

- Guide the representative's specific projects for measurable outcome.

- Review and document sales achievements.

- Comment on specific physician calls made during the trip.

- Discuss representative organizational skills, attitude.

- And, countless other observed representative behaviors.

Used as the management communication/documentation tool and report it was intended to be, the representative trip report can be an invaluable reference. It can be used to place a representative on probation or to terminate a representative, and your trip report scoring must be reflected in the Representative's counseling/appraisal evaluation session. To write one thing on a trip report and another on a counseling/appraisal and evaluation form is inviting disaster.

We feel accurate in saying, and confident in our belief, that if managers did a better job of documenting observed representative activity on working trips, far, far fewer cases would appear in front of the company's human resources and legal departments. *"If it isn't in writing, it didn't happen"* has been echoed many, many times in meetings with HR personnel.

So…how do you write a representative trip report, what should you observe on working trips, how do you establish working trip objectives for the Representative? How do you tailor trip objectives to individual representative? How do you discuss and review the work trip, at the end of the work trip, with the representative?

The next Work Trip. It is recommended to start this process informally on the first morning with a quick review of previous Work Trips.

Let's start this discussion of RTR's with how does one go about writing a trip report? We highly recommend that you write RTR's in the 2nd person referring to the representative as 'you'…the 2nd person keeps the report, as intended, as a personal report. 3rd person 'he or she' is too distant, and has the feeling of a cop writing up an accident report… *"the driver, he failed to make a proper turn and we need to arrest him"*. Use of 2nd person makes it feel as if you were there [which you were] and not a mere bystander reporting on activities. For example, *"**you** did an excellent job of scheduling **your** day…"*.

We can't emphasize enough the importance of setting tailor-made, individual RTR objectives. We recommend setting 2-3 objectives per work trip.

One of the Work Trip objectives should include a developmental skill you are working with the Rep on as a long-range project or goal as opposed to a Work Trip objective established specifically for one particular Work Trip. For example, if a Rep needs improvement on using a company approved medical journal article/reprint in a short, stand-up detail, and you are working with him on improving his ability to use reprints with physicians when time is short, one of the trip report objectives would be *To review/discuss how to use the "New England Journal of Medicine" article with physicians and to observe your use of the New England J Med article with 3-physicians on this Work Trip"*. This objective should be measurable by both rep and DM.

A 2nd Work Trip objective, if you have assigned individual, specific projects to each Rep in your District, would be to follow up on project progress on the Work Trip. For example, the Work Trip objective might be, "to review/discuss progress on getting 'X' formulary approved at the University of Colorado Health Science Center" or "to review/discuss progress on obtaining a speaker on 'x' date for the dinner-speaker program at the Hilton". Or... *"to discuss your territory 'working order' and make changes where necessary"*. Each trip report should refer to progress on previously set objectives, not a stand-alone document.

A third Working Trip objective, and one which gets you directly involved in the Rep's territory, is to <u>review specific sales objectives</u>. You do need to be careful with this objective and review because sales don't change that quickly from Work Trip to Work Trip, and you do not want to come across as being a detective or carrying a club. I once witnessed a 'scene' in a restaurant in Champaign, IL where a Pharmaceutical District Sales Mgr. used sales figures as a *'club'*, and it was anything but pretty...no recommendations from the manager on how to improve, no objectives or goal setting, just pounding on the Rep. Instead of looking for areas of improvement, and listening to the Rep relative to his problems/opportunities, this conversation was an ugly one-sided affair where nobody wins.

Many company Trip Reports have a section of the Trip Report devoted to sales and sales objectives, and this is good. If the Trip Report you are presently using does not have a section of the Trip Report devoted to a section allowing for comments on sales, then we would recommend that you set 'sales review' as a Work Trip objective.

Focus your attention during the Work Trip on the Work Trip Objectives you established when you last worked with the Representative. For example, if you are observing progress on using the *New England J Med* article in stand-up details, focus on this activity. Prior to the Work Trip you should have instructed the Rep to make as many calls as possible allowing the Rep to use the *New England J Med* article.

Carry a notebook along with you to make notes following calls. We don't recommend taking notes in front of the Rep [you look like a detective]. We do recommend jotting down a physician's name and call observations. You can excuse yourself from the Rep to do this. Another approach is to request a copy of today's planned work trip with individual call objectives. Brief notes can be put there after you step away. You should discuss progress as soon as possible following each call so there are really no surprises when you sit down with the Rep at the end of the Work Trip to write the Trip Report.

In writing up the RTR, you will want to use specific examples and specific physician names. For example, "you called on Dr Huggabone and..(what happened). Indicate what went well on the Rep's call on Dr Huggabone and any specific areas that need improvement that you noted in the Rep's call. We would highly recommend eliminating the word *"but"* from your Trip Report and Manager vocabulary in discussions with your Reps, and substitute in its place the word *"and"*. You can say 1,000-positive things, however, as soon as the *'but'* word appears, the Rep only hears what follows *'but'*. Involve the Rep in what went well and areas in which continued improvement or development may be needed. You want to comment on both in your Trip Report. You also want to spend time discussing work trip objectives for your next working trip with the Rep, and, schedule the time when you will next work together.

Your overall objective as a Manager is to instill confidence and trust. You are there for one purpose and that is to help the Rep [*"your customer"*] achieve his/her immediate and long-range business objectives. You want to instill trust that you and the Rep are working together as a team on all calls the Rep makes on his customers. Above all, be consistent in how you write Trip Reports and your behavior while on Work Trips.

We are of the belief that Trip Reports and Days-In-The-Field are critical to the Rep's success, and your success as a manager. RTR's set the tone for your relationship with the Rep and the over-all tone and direction for your District. Almost every management skill comes into play on a Rep Work Trip---communication, leadership, coaching, counseling, appraisal, observation, listening, team building and decision-making. And, after talking to many, many front-line District Sales Managers over the years, we have learned and concluded that the time you spend in the field with your Reps, and the writing of the Rep Trip Report, are paramount to your success as a manager. Focused teamwork over time between rep and manager can result in the Rep's ability to write future goals for themselves!

And, remember that, despite a stack of '*to do's*' sitting on your desk that need attention while you are working with one of your Reps in the field, we have never heard a Rep praise a manager for taking good, quality desk-time.

REPRESENTATIVE TRIP REPORTS

Opportunities

- *PRAISE* Rep performance – always start here!
- *DOCUMENT* areas in need of improvement.
- *GUIDE* Rep specific projects.
- Review/document sales achievements.
- Comment on specific calls.
- Coach.
- Discuss organization, attitude, etc.

REPRESENTATIVE TRIP REPORTS

Invaluable Reference

- Probation
- Termination
- Promotion
- Counseling and Appraisal
- Document/Document…and the HR Door

REPRESENTATIVE TRIP REPORTS

- Writing the Rep Trip Report *WITH* The Rep

- First morning…review previous and present RTP objectives

- Write report in 2nd Person

- Set tailor-made, specific, individual RTR objectives

REPRESENTATIVE TRIP REPORTS

Writing RTR objectives:

- "To review/discuss how to use the NEJM journal article with physicians and observe your use of the NEJM with 3-physicians in your territory".

- "To review/discuss progress on getting 'X' formulary approved at the University of Colorado Health Science Center".

- "To discuss your territory working order and make changes where necessary".

- "To review sales vs. objectives".

REPRESENTATIVE TRIP REPORTS

- Focus work trip and RTR on established RTR objectives.

- Carry a small Notebook.

- Don't Be A Detective.

- Remove the word 'but'.

- Install confidence and trust.

REPRESENTATIVE TRIP REPORTS

- Days-In-The-Field=Your Success Depends Upon It.

- We know of no single more important manager tool.

- RTR's set the tone, the mood and the outlook for the individual Rep and the entire District.

REPRESENTATIVE TRIP REPORTS

Case study...

- Experienced representative; average performer.

- 3rd time you have worked with him in this 'section' (Columbia) of his territory.

- You last worked the Columbia section with him 3-4 months ago.

- The Columbia section has the greatest number of physician's in Rep's territory.

- Representative took you to see the same physicians on this work trip as he did the last time you worked Columbia section with him.

- You did not document seeing the same physicians on the RTP the last time you worked the Columbia section with the Rep.

Questions

- Do you document this on the Trip Report? If so, how do you document?

- When do you return to this section?

- What do you say to the Rep? How do you approach?

REPRESENTATIVE TRIP REPORT

Case study...

- New Representative; you hired him.

- 3rd time you have worked with him.

- Around 4pm on the first day you work with him you note him looking at his watch; "did you have some paperwork you wanted to go over?"

- Around 4pm on the 2nd day…"do we need time to write-up the trip report"?

Questions

- What would you discuss with the Rep? How do you approach?

- What would you document?

- How would you write the trip report?

- What do you make as a RTR objective for the next time you work together?

REPRESENTATIVE TRIP REPORT

Case Study

- Experienced Rep; Columbia section.

- 3-months later, you are back working with the Rep in the Columbia section of his territory.

- RTR objectives state for the Rep to call on the following doctors in the Columbia section…Dr Huggabone, Dr Miller, Dr Marcus, Dr Nightingale.

- The Rep takes you on the same 'milk-run', i.e., sees same doctors

- Tries to see doctors Huggabone, Miller et al., and had the wrong time…"doctor sees reps at 5pm"…Rep called on doctor at noon.

Questions?

- How do you document?

- What do you do?

CHAPTER THREE
PLANNING AND ORGANIZATION

PLANNING & TIME MANAGEMENT

Planning is all about space and time. Don't be concerned that I'm going to move on to a discussion of Stephen Hawkings' theories, nothing as esoteric as that! Although man has probably wrestled with the twin concepts of space and time since he/she first gained an awareness of self.

You, as a manager, occupy space and you need time to get the things done that give you a sense of accomplishment in your work...in your career, for that matter. This sense of accomplishment is very important. You're likely throughout your career to get less recognition, *"thank you's, and "high fives"* than you truly deserve. So you need to construct your own recipe for accomplishment that will provide you self-fulfillment. In this way you sustain not only your self-esteem, but as important, your enjoyment of employment.

In our discussions with successful managers, that is - managers who have fielded teams that exceed quota and expectations while developing individuals to take on greater responsibility in the organization, we have found a consistent thread that ties them together. That thread is what I would characterize as a *passion* for being in the field working with the Representative. They will, when times demand, *"Rob Peter to pay Paul"*, so to speak, in order to gain that extra field time.

"*Robbing Peter to pay Paul*" can take many forms or avenues; for instance:

negotiating a due date with your boss over a report. If not needed ASAP, could it be worked into evening time, over-the-road, instead of canceling a field trip for more desk time. Boss says he wants to work with you next week. Next week you planned to be in Bismarck and Fargo. Would the following week work out OK, since you would be working with Reps that are closer to home, so that there is less travel and down time? Invest extra effort to assure that isolated reps receive the same visit time as your closely located reps.

Many sales organizations have found that, for a front-line field manager, a staff of ten Representatives is a good balance between span of control and a life beyond work. There has been a move in the last generation within organizations to load more and more onto the front-line field manager while expecting less and less desk time in return. This initiative has been found to be very damaging. The manager's life gets out of balance. Stress enters the picture doing damage both spiritually and physically not only to the manager, but also to those that are dependent on the manager for leadership. Managers need to oppose and question this tendency if they see it happening to them… oppose individually by addressing the problem with their boss and as a group at manager meetings with the hierarchy.

How important is planning and time management to how you will accomplish what you will accomplish as managers? Here is what Harold McAlindon has to say…"*Planning is 80% thinking and 20% writing. Then 100% doing!*" This segues nicely with Thomas Edison's response to his success as an inventor. "*It's 90% perspiration and 10% inspiration.*" Put them together and you are in for a lot of inspired thinking.

Where to begin? I tend to attack the challenge of planning spatially within a time frame. What do we have readily available as a graphic and visual tool that combines both? You've guessed it…A Month-At-A-Glance Calendar on your laptop or notebook or smart phone. The overall objective as a front-line manager, for me, was to gain as many "four days in the field and one day at desk" weeks as possible within the fiscal year. It is a continuous and ever-changing process that requires gamesmanship. There will be days in the weeks and weeks in the year that you are out of the field for other commitments. Block these out of field days on your calendar (in pencil) be they for manager con-

ferences, sales meetings, training conferences, recruiting and interviewing…
or whatever. I call it *"planning with a laptop"* because inevitably there will
be changes, postponements, even cancellations. Change is the only constant
here.

There is another constant we all must deal when it comes to Desk Days. And
that is that there is never enough *"day"* in *Desk Day!* One day a week seems to
be an inadequate amount of time to address and manage all the tasks and "have
to(s)" that have been stored up over the week. In the past it was primarily
paper (mail) and phone calls (and notes from phone calls). Now you contend
with not only the U.S. Mail, perhaps of greater volume, the E-mails along with
fax(s) and stored phone mail text messages. In this age of portable computers,
you have the ability to organize tasks on the run, so to speak, and determine
which to save for your office day and which to address over the course of your
days and evenings in the field.

One caution to interject here regarding the mixing of *"office time" with "field
time"*. When you are working with your Representative *"in the field"*, you
really need to demonstrate with that individual that he/she has your full and
undivided attention. You are there for them. However, with the reality of
limited access in some areas of hospitals and clinics, where the Representative
must tread lightly and having a manager tagging along just complicates and
restricts performance, you may give the most realistic support by hanging out
in the lobby or waiting room during the course of that sales call. That's a
time when you can decant phone mail messages and/or work on tasks that you
have stored in your laptop/notebook. It is also a time that you can make some
notes on how the day is going with the particular Rep with some specifics on
previous calls made in preparation for the sit-down over the Rep Trip Report.

So here you are at your desk on your **Desk Day**. Where to begin?

The <u>first task</u> is collecting and collating the tasks by time frame (due date) and
importance (priority).

I've found over the years that the very low tech *"piles method"* is a fair start.
This method relies on your ability *to "pile"* the email by subject and due date.
File only that which you wish to bury for unlikely reference at a later date. As
regards files, I have found that an overall segmenting into broad subject areas
works well.

These <u>broad subject areas</u> could take the title(s):

- Home Office Administration.

- Administrative Forms.

- Field Administration, Rep

   - Salary/compensation

   - District/Division Sales vs. Quotas

   - Field Operations Manual

   - H.R./Legal.

- Personal Files, Rep Travel Files.

- Manager Personal Files.

- Directories & Addresses.

- Projects & Assignments.

- "Ongoing Correspondence" and

- Miscellaneous.

CHAPTER FOUR
COMMUNICATION

COMMUNICATION...UP, DOWN AND SIDEWAYS

"Three things in life do not come back...and one of them is the spoken word"
Anonymous.

The one managerial trait, above all other managerial traits, which we have observed over the course of our careers, that separates the effective manager from the average manager, is the ability to communicate. Why are some managers better communicators than other managers? What does it take to be an effective communicator? Why do some Districts and Regions thrive on communication while in other Districts and Regions, nary a word is spoken or written?

Communication begins with the manager. The more you, as the manager, encourage communication between you and your Representatives, the more communication you will receive. The more enthusiastic you are about communication and communicating up and down, the more enthusiastic the people you work with become about communication. If you want to develop 'open' lines of communication with your team (and with your boss), work hard on fostering a spirit of communication...that you thrive on communication. We have observed, reported to and listened to a number of managers over the years that follow the communication philosophy of "just send me the important stuff". Unfortunately, communication doesn't work like that. It is not up to the 'sender' to decide what is important to the *'reader'*. And, most importantly, while some communication is *'nice to know'*, communication is a 'building' process. It is taking little bits of information at a time and building on the information.

The **keys to communication**, both written and oral, are:

- Communication needs to be continuous---your channels of communication need to be 'open' at all times. You can't feel like communicating some days and not others. You must be 'tuned in' at all times. Your goal is to respond within 24-hours.

- *"Live-Line"* communication---we can't stress enough having a list of topics you wish to discuss written out ahead of the telephone call, taking notes on the call, filing your notes and, most importantly, coming to an agreement with the person you are talking to relative to a 'plan of action'.

- *"I'm glad you called", "thanks for the voicemail", "thanks for taking the time to send me an e-mail on"*---your Representatives must feel good about communicating with you and that you are genuinely interested in what they have to tell you. Enthusiasm is the key in all of your communication. Respond and reply with positive specifics.

- Clear, succinct and to the point---in all communications, get to the point quickly and make sure your reader understands exactly what message you are conveying

- Listening---you can't be a good communicator without the ability to listen. There have been 1,000's of books written on listening and how to improve your listening skills.

- The two listening skills we feel most important---

  o (i) let the person finish what he/she has to say.

  o (ii) don't anticipate ahead of time what you think the person is going to say. Do ask questions for a clearer understanding.

CELL PHONE AND EMAIL

Cell phone direct telephone communication

Some managers set up scheduled, planned weekly calls with each rep.

Have a list of topics you wish to discuss written out ahead of the telephone call.

Are you calling at a convenient time?

Take notes on the call.

File your notes immediately after the call.

Come to an agreement with the person you are talking to relative to an agreed upon 'plan of action'.

Thank the person you are talking to for taking time to talk to you.

Voicemail

While guidelines for using cell phones should be established, we recommend keeping them general in nature so as not to discourage communication; too many rules/regulations discourage communication.

We recommend your using a cell phone for short messages which require immediate action of the receiver.

If you must leave an instructional cell phone message, tell your listener that you will follow up the message with an email memo or written communication.

Remember---more information is misinterpreted when sent via cell phone than any other method of communication.

Texting with Smart Phones –

First, be aware that the first word in the subject line is most important.

Be meticulous in your brief message, as auto-correct and missing correct letters can truly change your message.

Always read your message before you hit 'send'.

If you are requesting some action from the rep, that request should be first, not buried in the message.

Email and Letters/Memos

We highly recommend that you communicate via electronic mail with one topic per email.

Indicate the 'subject' of your email carefully…this will help the reader file the email if necessary. If there is a due date for reply, that goes at the top.

Outline the purpose of your e-mail memo up front and get to the point quickly and succinctly.

Use 'bullet' points whenever possible.

Remember the Human Resources axiom…*"if it isn't in writing, it doesn't exist"*.

Hand-Written Notes

Anytime you wish to recognize a job well done by one of your Representatives or anytime you wish to thank someone for their effort, we highly recommend that you do so on via a hand-written, signed note mailed directly to whom you are writing.

"The Elements of Style" by Strunk -- the one book we would highly recommend above all others to learn about writing skills.

Communicating With Your Boss

Put it in writing.

Avoid lengthy cell phone messages, and especially those which require receiver to take notes.

Always follow up cell phone messages with a written note or email.

As with all communication, state your purpose and outline your thoughts so the reader can follow what you have to say.

Build a 'tickle file' of the achievements of each rep, and their areas to improve.

The Art of Communication

Encourage communication on:

Sales ideas.

Success stories.

What the competition is saying and doing.

New medical journal articles on your drug or competitive drugs.

Problem-solving.

"There is no limit to how far a man can go or what he can do if he does not mind who gets the credit" ____sign posted in President Ronald Reagan's White House office.

Knowledge is power and communication is the means in which knowledge is passed from one person to another. There has been a lot said over the years on the subject of what information to share and communicate with the Representative.

Q. Why do some Districts and Regions communicate better than others?

A. Because the manager encourages communication and gives thanks for receiving.

Communication and team building go 'hand-in-hand'.

Nice-to-know information can quickly turn to important-to-know…read and listen carefully to all of your communications.

Remember…as the Manager, <u>you set the tone</u> and the stage for all communications with the Representatives you are supervising. Communication is a 2-way street. Provide quality communication out and quality communication comes back your way.

CHAPTER SIX
ADJUSTING FROM REP TO MANAGER

FROM REPRESENTATIVE TO MANAGER...MAKING THE CHANGE

"We should get out of an experience the wisdom that is in it, and stop there. Otherwise, we will be like the cat that sits on a hot stove-lid. The cat will never sit on a hot stove-lid again, and that is well. But, the cat will never sit on a cold stove-lid either" —Mark Twain

In this section we provide our thoughts on making the change from Representative to Manager. We will focus on how to think and act like a manager, and outline some of the common problems in making the transition.

THINKING AND ACTING LIKE A MANAGER

A Brand New Manager---it is a lot easier to be *'strict'* at the start, and loosen up as you go, than to try to do it the other way around.

Expectations---we highly encourage setting expectations from the start---what you expect from your Representatives and what they can expect from you.

Rules/Regulations---we firmly believe in following the key management axiom of "ask me a business question, and I'll give you a business answer", and we think it prudent to know and to follow each company rule and policy carefully. We have seen more Managers run into trouble because they did not take the time to read/review, and be familiar with the Company's Procedure Manual for such things as vacation time, sick days, time off territory, personal leave, etc., etc.

Good Old Boys Club---like it or not, the title and the job of Manager separates you from the Representatives you are supervising. You are no longer a member of "the good old boys club"…so stay above the gossip and stay away from spending the night in a bar at a sales meeting with your Representatives. This is not to say you can't have a drink with your group. What we are saying here is that your Representatives need time and space, and it is a natural thing with all Representatives to be able to talk amongst themselves about their boss.

Being Liked…Being Respected---the decisions you make as a Manager are often very tough decisions, and may not be liked by all members of your District/Region. However, tough decisions are what you are getting paid to do. We would recommend concentrating your managerial decision-making efforts on being fair, consistent and open, thus gaining the respect of your group, rather than making decisions based on being liked by the group. We all want to be liked. Work hard on being consistent and fair and the respect will come…so will the like.

Patience…A Tough Lesson To Learn---one of the biggest surprises you will experience in working with your Representatives for the first, second or third time as a new Manager is the immediate realization that not all of your Representatives work (sell products) like you did. It can come as a shock. We think it is important to remember that every Representative has his/her own style. The point to be made is that it is important to take your time observing, and not to try to change things over night. It just can't be done and it leads to tremendous frustration. Build on the good in each Representative.

Personal Problems---a word to the wise…while we think it is important to be empathetic and caring relative to Rep's personal problems, and that you should take interest in a Rep's family, we encourage you to stay focused on the business side of being a manager, and let the Rep bring up personal matters to you. Talk and think business while you are working with your Representatives.

Managing Down---one of the first tendencies as a new Manager is to prove to everyone (especially your Boss) that you are a good Manager, and management's decision to put you in the position as Manager was a good one.

Because of this tendency to want to 'show your managerial stuff', there is an inclination, conscious or unconscious, to begin to 'manage up' toward your Boss. Your job is to manage the people you are responsible for...do a good job in managing these people [managing down, if you will, and the rest will take care of itself.

You Are On Display---remember, you are no longer a Representative, and every action you take is being observed by your Representatives. Leave a Representative at noon during a work trip, and the word gets out that the boss is cutting out at noon. Actions speak louder than words. The same holds true for communication...take 2-days to get back with a Representative, and you will shortly find that your team will take 2-or more days to get back with you.

Be You---at the start of a management career, there is a general tendency to emulate a boss or manager's style you liked. And, while there is nothing wrong with that, you are you, and being yourself is important from the start. The real you will come out over time anyway, so be yourself from the start. Concentrate at the start of your career on working on your weaknesses. For example, if you are a procrastinator, work on scheduling your time and getting what needs to be done. If you are disorganized, learn how to get organized. We personally feel organizational skills need to be learned from the start as more management time is wasted and problems occur through poor organization than any other single cause.

CHAPTER SEVEN
LEADERSHIP

LEADERSHIP! WHAT IS IT?

"If you don't throw it, they can't hit it" —Lefty Gomez

We have done a lot of reading on it and no one I can find has a good handle on *"What it is"* or *"What is it?"* It's kind of like that wet bar of soap, just as soon as you think you've got you hand around it and start to squeeze…Out it pops and slips below the surface!

Let's take a look at what is a likely scenario. You, a successful Representative, have just been promoted to Field Manager. Your new boss instills some confidence by stating that he/she knows you'll do well based on your previous record of accomplishment (Good!). Oh! And, in addition, you will be counted on to be a leader of your new sales team (Whoops!). Yesterday, you were a productive, successful Rep, and somehow, overnight, you were magically instilled into the mysteries, not only of sound management practices, but also the art of leadership. The use of the terms *"practices"* and *"art"* is intentional. Practices are more easily defined than is art. There's the rub! One person sees art that is not recognized as such by another. Art tends to be in the mind of the beholder.

Study of famous people who have been labeled great leaders is somewhat instructional.

Even here you can get in an argument pretty quickly over your pick as either "great" or "leader". I'll throw in a few to stir up the pot. Winston Churchill, FDR, Gandhi, A. Lincoln, Martin Luther King, Susan B. Anthony, Attila the Hun, Margaret Sanger, Harry Truman and Douglas MacArthur. Some might have trouble with Attila, yet a book has been written on his leadership *style*. Harry Truman and Douglas MacArthur form an interesting combo, since Harry as President went ahead and fired Doug as General of the Armies for insubordination (Considered by many to be a brave thing to do, given Mac's popularity). What is the similarity here? All of these individuals were just that…quite unique unto themselves. And all very complex with attributes that at times were strength and at other times weakness. Biographers have recorded how others have described Winston Churchill as *"inspirational"*, *"manipulative"*, *"courageous"*, *"maddening"*,

We don't seem to be getting too far using this approach. So, instead, I'm going to suggest we pose the query, "What do people value in one who might be their leader?" **How about…*Honest, Trustworthy, Trustful, Consistent, Respectful, Straight & Open, Empathetic, Forward looking, Risktaker, Inspiring, Expectant and Optimistic with a Sense of Humor.***

Over the years, thanks to some hard knocks and missteps along the way, I've formulated what we call ***Management Maxims***. These are rules of conduct I wish someone had given me when starting out as a brand new Field Manager. They begin the structure of *Field Driven Management©* and perhaps with application, timing and luck *Value Base Leadership©*. In the words of Oscar Wilde, *"Experience is the name everyone gives to their mistakes."*

SO HERE GOES...

MANAGEMENT MAXIMS

Establish expectations early on.

Conduct business in an ethical and professional manner.

Always be on time.

Ask how Rep wishes to be addressed. Be careful with ascribing nicknames.

Beware of the gray line that separates business from personal.

Be very sparing in advice given that is not business related.

Be a good listener and know the difference between empathy and sympathy.

Know that everything you do or say is being recorded by an observing Rep.

Be very selective in the use of humor, never at the other's expense.

Neither recognize nor encourage racial, religious or ethnic slurs or jokes.

Be frank and straight-forward. (Reps sniff out hidden agendas).

Be very careful when discussing money (raises and bonuses)…have your facts correct before you speak.

There is always, *always*, more than one side to a story.

You can't coach if you do not stay up with the sales materials…don't become a "babysitter".

Spend time with your top performers…learn from them.

Mistakes…you will make mistakes…learn from them.

Problems only get bigger with more time and wishing never makes them go away.

Check facts carefully and ask for help from the other person for understanding.

Encourage learning about your products and your competitor's products.

Complaints and criticism…if you have one, have a solution.

Work very hard to stay organized…so much time is wasted on trying to find things.

Whenever possible always provide options. (Don't back people into corners).

Recognize value and contributions. Sincere "*Thank you's*" are appreciated.

Celebrate success both individually and as a team.

Share information. Withholding does not lead to control, it engenders distrust.

Remember that one-way communication is fraught with potential for misunderstanding. Take responsibility for miscommunication.

Establish yourself as your team's contact with your regional and headquarters. This will keep you informed, and you can likely enhance any request that might have been made to HQ.

Deal with observed behavior and document.

"Ask me a business question; I'll give you a business answer".

Teambuilding does not start with staying out late at a sales meeting with your representatives at sales meetings.

Don't threaten. Instead explain consequences of actions and behavior.

Confront problems immediately.

Keep it positive and be enthusiastic…you set the tone and mood of the District.

Concentrate on strengths. Doing so often minimizes shortcomings and builds confidence.

Career promotions…from the Halleman School of Management - don't make a lot of false promises.

Representative trip report and sales objectives must be thought out very carefully before putting them in writing.

Remember, as a manager, <u>your success</u> is measured through the success of your Representatives as a team. It follows, therefore, that you are there for them.

LET'S TAKE A CLOSER LOOK AT A FEW OF THESE MAXIMS. THERE IS A STORY BEHIND EACH.

Establish expectations early on.

Getting on solid footing with the Representative right from the start will reduce initial stress and foster an open work environment. I remember starting out in my first career after college. I came aboard a large corporation that made jet engines. I worked as a technical writer in the Service Bulletin Group. No one sat down with me on day one to go over the ground rules or to establish what was expected from me. Had to figure it out on my own as best I could. Came up with 1. Don't be late for work.; 2. Don't ask for too much help.; 3. If you don't have anything to do, just try to look busy.; 4. Don't ask *"How am I doing?"* That would be rude! After a year I announced to the boss that I was leaving to go into pharmaceutical sales. He seemed surprised and a bit taken back. Said I had done good work and they were pleased with me. He had recently lost another relatively new employee who was thought highly of… and wondered why.

Ask how Rep wishes to be addressed. Be careful ascribing nicknames.

Some years ago, I worked a combined District Meeting with a peer from Chicago. He was in the habit of ascribing nicknames to all of his staff. I'm sure some really liked the practice, since it made them feel a part of the inside circle. I also know one who did not. His name was Tom, the manager called him "Tommy Joe". Although this Rep was a team player and smiled wanly, he seethed underneath as he saw it demeaning.

Neither recognize nor encourage racial, religious or ethnic slurs or jokes.

During a District Sales meeting a Representative who prided himself with always having information or an answer before anyone else chimed in that he had the answer to a question that came up about whether or not we would be supplied with a particular medical study/reprint for an upcoming product promotion. When I said I'd have to call Marketing to find out, he said he already had and we would! His name was Tom, a different Tom and he was Polish. One of the other Reps made an offhand remark that as Reps they were not supposed to call the office but instead go through the manager. He then connected this to a *"Dumb Pollack Joke"* and got a laugh from the audience. I ignored the comment and laughter and went on with the meeting. That night I got a call at home from a very upset Tom. How would you, as manager, respond in this situation?

Know that everything you do or say is being recorded by an observing Rep.

This Maxim is worth repeating to yourself before you begin each Day-In-The-Field with a Representative. Your commitment is required to set an example by behaving in ways that are consistent with shared values…or what can become shared values. As you value the individual so will that individual value you. As you value your responsibilities so will that individual value their responsibilities. As you value your company so will that individual value your Company and make it *their* company. A leader models his/her behavior so that he/she can be looked to for leadership. Even though this is defining something by itself, it is still true and right. Leaders have a continuing awareness that their behavior and deportment inspire those around them who are seeking a leader to guide them.

VALUE DRIVEN LEADERS…

model the way

share Core Values

project and reflect optimism

articulate a mission

use visualization as a driver

seek common purpose

stay the course

exhibit humanity

CHAPTER EIGHT
TEAM BUILDING

TEAM BUILDING...DEVELOPING A WINNING TEAM

"To be a good hitter, you've got to get a good pitch to hit" —Ted Williams

We have observed over the years, and we think it is due to the nature of the job itself and the personality traits of individuals who do the job, the need on the part of pharmaceutical sales representatives to belong and feel part of a group or team. In this section we'll examine ways for you to develop a team, how to keep the team 'feeling' going forward and why teambuilding is an important aspect of management. Building a team just doesn't happen; it takes a lot of continuous work on the manager's part. Team building has emphasis on the 'building'...you are always building.

The need to belong and the need to be part of a group are strong needs of the pharmaceutical sales representative. While not psychology experts, we believe the need exists with pharmaceutical representatives because the job, for the most part, is an independent one, e.g., you don't work in an office where there are a lot of people. Basically, in pharmaceutical sales, one works independently of others. You have your own physician call list, your own geographical boundaries, etc. So the need to belong is there.

Coupled with the need to belong is the need for peer recognition. The need for approval and recognition is stronger in pharmaceutical sales than most managers imagine. Countless representative interviews over the years have highlighted the fact that one thing that builds a strong, cohesive, all-for-one, one-for-all team is recognition. The road to building a good team is paved with recognizing individual and group accomplishments and efforts on an on-going basis.

DEVELOPING A DISTRICT/REGION TEAM NAME & SLOGAN/MOTTO

We think the road to building a team begins with developing a team name, motto and slogan. If your District/Region does not have a name, we suggest talking to your Representatives and have a mini-contest to come

up with the best name for the team. Geography can be important in a team name, e.g., The Western Stars or the Chicago Whirlwinds, but we have seen District/Region team names developed from the manager's name. For example, District Sales Manager Joe Hecker's District team name was *"Hecker's Heroes"*.

Whatever District/Region name the group decides upon, you will want to put the team name on all District/Region Sales Bulletins and use the name whenever possible on group email messages.

We also strongly suggest that, in addition to a team name, you and the group develop a motto or slogan for the team. For example, *"The Western Stars… The Relentless Pursuit of Perfection"*. A slogan or motto gives your group a common, shared vision. It is the future vision that you want to develop…a shared goal, if you will.

Consider establishing a district "rapid response call sequence" so you only call one or two reps to start the call, and your team will follow thru with the rest.

FOSTERING TEAM SPIRIT

District/Region Sales Bulletins---there is, in our opinion, no better way to foster team spirit than through Sales Bulletins/Memos that feature the team name and slogan. We would also encourage you to develop some type of logo to use on the Sales Bulletin. For example, a lightning bolt, star or picture of a tornado can add a lot to the concept you are trying to develop. Also, we would encourage putting an inspirational quote at the beginning or end of each District Sales Bulletin.

District/Region Sales Meetings---there is no better time when the group comes together to promote the feeling of team spirit. PowerPoint slides used in presenting information to the group should have the team name or logo on them. Bring a sign for your meeting room as well.

Representative Working Trips---on work trips

with Representatives in your District or Region, you want to make every effort to speak highly of the team's accomplishments and how proud you are of the success. If done carefully, and not overdone, mentioning other team member success stories on working trips can foster the spirit of everyone pulling together.

COMMUNICATION...THE KEY TO SUCCESSFUL TEAM BUILDING

Enthusiasm---there is no tool in your sales manager's briefcase that has more impact on a group than your expressed genuine enthusiasm.

Recognition---time after time in Representative surveys of how their manager is doing, the one downfall mentioned over 95% of the time is that the manager does not spend enough time recognizing and communicating Representative successes. You may think you are doing a good job of recognizing individual and group successes, and what opinion surveys show is that you need to double your present recognition communication just to be at an effective level. The harder you work at recognizing your team's successes, the more team successes you will see. Communicate success. Look for success.

"How Are We Doing?"---every member of your team is interested in his team's performance and how the team is doing against other teams. As a District Manager in St Louis, the District Manager in Louisville and I ran two or three District contests per year, complete with weekly scoreboards...the camaraderie and team building was tremendous. The same holds true for District sales scoreboards outlining how your District/Region is doing compared to other Districts/Regions. Competition builds team spirit. There is a reason they keep baseball standings. *"It's Your Show"*---while communication develops spirit, which develops team attitude, it is the manager's job to communicate a vision of looking at the positive. Nothing is more demoralizing to a Team than to hear a manager say a few positive things about the group's accomplishments, only to turn the next statement into a *'but'*, e.g., you did all of these things well, *'but'*...communicate positively.

TEAM BUILDING...SOME FINAL THOUGHTS

Working With A Representative In The Field---we have always been of the belief that you want to develop on an individual basis with each Representative, that when you make joint calls together on physicians, nurses, pharmacists or other customers, that you go in together as a 'team'. You are the manager, and as the manager, it is your job to evaluate performance, and we think performance is best served by communicating with each Representative your desire to work as a team in calling on customers. If a prescriber asks why you should accompany the rep in the office, a good reply is, *"So I can see what a great job my rep is doing"*.

Bad-Mouthing Team Members---it should go without saying that when working with one Representative that you should always avoid bad-mouthing the performance of another Representative in your District or Region. Nothing kills team building (or confidence and trust for that matter) than a manager who goes around his/her District bad-mouthing Representatives behind their backs. Always keep it positive.

"Keep It Simple, Be Practical and Get A Raise"---in all communications, remember to keep it simple and positive. While team building takes time, and will not be accomplished overnight, your goal as a manager is to take pride in your team and express it every way possible. Keep track of what Representatives in your District/Region are doing, and communicate those successes as frequently as possible. I used to publish a District *"The Year In Review"* bulletin outlining individual Rep accomplishments and highlights which was well received by the Team.

If You Have Trouble---saying *"nice job'* or *"well done'*, and a surprisingly high number of managers simply can't utter the words *"good job"*, then we highly recommend you work hard at changing and force yourself to recognize success. For it has been our experience that the managers who consistently score low on management ability surveys, do not recognize success. The interesting thing is this…a manager could be an administrative wiz, handle problems effectively and punctually, be organized to the max, etc., etc.…, and be labeled a 'bad manager' for the simple reason that they are not giving Representatives what the vast majority need, and that is recognition.

Final Thoughts…if you want to develop a team, the team needs to feel the following:

- The Team Captain (you) are there for them.

- You are managing your customers (your Representatives) and not managing up to get your next promotion.

- You aren't turning 'trust' into a 4-letter word.

- No matter who comes up with the sales idea that is passed up-the-line and recognized----you, you and the Representative or the Representative, it is always the Representatives idea when the idea is passed up. You always give credit to the Representative [or your customer], especially with your manager.

- A good goal is to prepare your reps for promotion by giving them special assignments, such as presenting a subject at a district meeting.

"BE MORE ASSERTIVE!"…SOME THOUGHTS

Perhaps you've heard this exclamation from someone as advice for greater success in selling.

What does it mean? Might well ask the advice giver for more direction. Perhaps the advice giver is not all that articulate in defining just what "assertiveness" is or is not.

Over the years I have read books and listened to tapes on the subject of "*assertiveness*". Even the so-called experts don't line up in agreement.

What is assertiveness not? It is neither aggressiveness nor combativeness. It is not manipulative. It is not *"getting your way"* at the expense of others. It is not *"Win-Lose"*.

So what is *"assertiveness"*? Simply put, it is letting others know what you would like (to happen or have happen)... That's all. It is being *"up front"* with people. So how does this relate to sales? Think about it. What is more irksome than to be having a conversation with someone, knowing that they want something, but not being able to guess what that something is?

There is a *"best practices"* way of going about this. It follows techniques shown to be successful in a sales situation. Basically, you first gain an interchange on what may support your request for what you would like. You create a climate for an exchange of ideas to allow the other person to have their say and state opinion. Summarize the key points and then ask with the understanding that the other individual has your permission and the freedom to say *"No!"*.

A *"No!"*, should it happen, isn't the end of the world nor probably the end of the dialogue. It establishes a basis for further discussion and negotiation. It is not based on the emotions of fear or anger. It is not a stressful situation. It is based on clear thought and reasoning. It is likely to result in a *"Win-Win"* outcome or at least a reasonable compromise. By the way... this all works as well in relating to anyone, be it prescriber or a business associate,

CHAPTER TEN
COACHING & COUNSELING

❝❝People don't ask for facts in making up their minds. They would rather have one good, soul-satisfying emotion than a dozen facts" Robert Leavitt

We have observed over the years a number of managerial traits which make a manager a successful coach and counselor. The purpose of this section is to review some of the characteristics of successful coaches/counselors and provide you with a roadmap of how to work on, and continue to improve, your coaching and counseling skills.

CHARACTERISTICS OF SUCCESSFUL COACHES/COUNSELORS:

Listen Like Your Job Depended Upon It---one of the key characteristics or traits of a successful coach/counselor, and considered by many to be the single most important trait, is the **ability to listen**. The ability to listen carefully to not only what the person is saying, but the ability of not pre-judging what is being said, guessing what the person is going to say before they say it or letting your mind wander while the individual is talking. Countless books have been written on listening, and basically they all say the same thing…to be a good listener, you need to focus on what the person is saying as if the words were the last words the person was ever going to say, not upon your next response. Time after time in surveys Reps complete on what they like best about their manager, the words "*he is a good listener*" are always near the top of the list.

Understanding---coupled with listening, a successful coach/counselor needs to be able to understand and identify what it is that the person is trying to say. Phrases like *"what I hear you saying"* and repeating a key spoken phrase for clarity are traits of successful coaches.

You Need Not Know All the Answers---many times, new managers feel that they have to know and be able to make a decision on every question that is fired their way from their Representatives. Successful coaches/counselors are always in the *'learning mode'* and *'open'* to what the subordinate or peer have to say about a problem or situation. You need not know everything. Nor do you need to make a snap decision on everything. You do need to be 'open' and flexible in your thinking. And, you need to admit that you don't know everything.

Stick To The Issues---if you are coaching a Rep on how to use reprints during a sales presentation, we encourage you to remember to stick to the issue of using a reprint…don't get off on tangents like closing the sale, how to ask the right questions or other things. Therefore, it is important to have an idea of what it is you want to coach/counsel ahead of time.

Coach On Strengths---one of the key characteristics of successful coaches is the ability to build on an individual's strengths. If you want to motivate some-one to do something or to improve, for example, a sales skill, it is important to point out what the individual is already doing correctly. People want to do the right thing and be successful. Your job as a coach is to strengthen their belief that they are doing the right thing and are doing a good job.

"Well managed, motivated organizations give their people the right to be wrong" —Laurel Cutler

Timing Is Essential---successful coaches/counselors coach immediately following the event or situation…don't wait till the end of the day to start coaching.

The Word Is Sincere---it goes without saying that successful coaches gen-uinely care about the person they are coaching. They are taking the time to coach/counsel because they want their Representative to be successful. If you turn 'trust' into a 4-letter word, you will not be a successful coach.

Earning Respect---to be a successful coach/counselor, you have to be respected. You gain respect through communication and trust.

Coaching Versus Dictating---there is, and always will be, a fine line between coaching/counseling and ordering people to do something. "You must do this" isn't coaching. *"You might consider trying"* is coaching. Asking "How would you approach this" is seeking input for a solution.

Experience---you will become a better coach, counselor and teacher with experience. . The important thing about being a good coach is to continually work at developing a level of communication with both your new Reps and your experienced Reps. It is the art of communication...what to say and when that makes a successful coach.

Counseling---a couple of thoughts on the Counseling & Appraisal process. First, when you sit down with your Representatives to conduct their annual or semi-annual counseling and appraisal sessions it is critical to remember that in your performance review there should be no major surprises. The session should consist of an exchange of information and a review/summary of the information you have discussed with each Rep throughout the year or throughout the performance evaluation period. Trust becomes a 4-letter word when you surprise someone with a rating that totally comes from 'left' field.

Second, we think it is important during the C&A session to let each Representative know where they stand in the District...top quarter, top half, etc., and what the Rep needs to do to move up in the District rankings.

Counseling & Appraisal Sessions---we would highly encourage you to send the C&A form to the Rep prior to the evaluation session to allow the Rep a chance to make comments under each section of the evaluation form. This offers the Rep the opportunity to voice his/her comments and feel that he/she had a say in the process. It also allows for an excellent exchange during the C&A session.

Enthusiasm---a successful coach displays genuine enthusiasm when one of his Representatives scores a success.

A Vision---develop a vision for your Team. Nothing pulls a group together like a shared vision. *"The true motivation for employees is the spirit of cooperation that comes with a shared vision"* ____Greg Bustin

Coaching The New and the Experienced Rep---while the new and the experienced Rep need praise and need to be appreciated the same, in today's market, based on interviews with new and experienced Reps, we note that it is very important to spend time coaching new Representatives [more so than experienced Representatives] on how to increase their chances of seeing the tough-to-see physician. Rejection is one of the top reasons new representatives leave pharmaceutical sales. We would also highly recommend coaching your new and experienced Reps on how to sell physicians when time is short and during stand-up details. We reviewed and discussed both of these situations in-depth in our new book *"How To Sell Pharmaceuticals And Medical Devices When You Are Really Not Sue How"*. The book is available on sheeleyconsulting.com. We would highly recommend this book as it discusses in detail how to get a provider to use a drug for the first time. The important concept of "patient-type centered selling"© is discussed.

DEVELOPING PLANS FOR IMPROVEMENT

Representative trip reports, counselling after calls and at the end of working trips are the vital front line of establishing a great working relationship not only with each rep in your district, but with your team as a group.

It is vital that you have established your expectations very early on, and they may include frequency of visits to zip codes and to each category of prescriber. You may have territory reports that you request as well. Timely and accurate submissions of expense reports are vital as you must approve each one and forward approvals to HQ. Have your team members planned their working orders with a copy to you? It is also good to request that you be informed of any new challenges that any team member encounters. Be sure you have communicated clearly about these aspects of working in your district. You can't help your team with things you don't know about. Establish that if they have any reason to contact HQ or your regional manager, they should go thru you. You are there for them, and likely can help find a way to satisfy a request.

Nota Bene: When you send an email that requests an action or reply to you, place that fact at the <u>very top</u> of your email, so that everyone will know when a reply is due, and what is to be included in the reply.

The first two words of your email Subject Line are critical, as that is all some smart phones display and it helps your team know the importance of requested due dates.

No matter how carefully you have conducted your interviews and hiring, there will be rare occasions when a given representative is not performing the many duties of a position up to your team standards. Careful planning of your field trip goals with this representative, followed by factual documentation in your field trip report is the first step. You have the goal of modifying the representative's performance so that they can move forward with the rest of the district. Start with positives you have observed and document them along with agreed upon things to improve with specific, measurable parameters that you carefully document. If you are not seeing improvement, you need to gather insight and support for your next step by first contacting your Regional Manager with an analysis that displays your concern and efforts to date. Your RM may suggest either a meeting with all other DM's in the region, or recommend one or two for you to contact for their insight about how to proceed. Your RM will likely request you to file a report with HR.

Medical Sales positions are highly detail oriented and since you have had the Rep position, you know where some corners may be cut, so it should be very unlikely a rep could pull the wool over your eyes for an extended period of time.

Here are some aspects that you may focus upon to document where changes need to be made:

- Calls may be reported that are not sampled, so no signature would be required, thus fairly easy to add calls that were not made.

- Sampling Signed call cards are kept in HQ, and those signatures can be compared over time.

- Post Call notes need to be specific, including the call goal, what was discussed, what the response was, and what the plan will be for the next visit.

- Post Call notes should therefore be individualized, not all the same.

- Office data should be up to date, with best times to visit, and names of key office staff.

- Company Car mileage should be recorded at the end of each day, separated into personal mileage and business mileage per corporate guidelines.

- Expense account receipts for meals, and overnights, should be dated and within allowable spend limits.

- Meals and overnights should be within the pre-planned territory rotation unless there is an exception that you were made aware of.

- Gasoline receipts should parallel the distance and dates from home to those working zip codes, with listed daily mileage fitting in smoothly.

- Your RM may have access to documentation for any new traffic tickets with the company car.

- Vehicle maintenance such as oil changes and tire rotations should be made in a timely manner.

- Territory call efforts should be focused primarily upon the most valuable prescribers, you can use your printout of their targets to inquire about what the rep has tried, starting at the top of their list.

You may be asked to develop a Plan for Improvement for that representative. Your approach to the rep could be very important towards maintaining team morale. How you handle this can demonstrate that you have their backs while expecting them to individually work hard to maintain your support as a team effort.

Towards the end of your introduction and discussion of the Plan for Improvement, noting specifics and perhaps a sequence of due dates, **ask the rep how they will make the changes come about.** Importantly, this is not your statement of how you would handle this, you want to know what they believe will work for them. Tell them that you will happily note progressive changes as they apply their full effort going forward.

CHAPTER ELEVEN
CASES

MANAGEMENT CASES

- Due to physician growth and/or a new product launch, you need to realign territories. One particular territory has a high percentage of ivory-tower, consultant type physicians who get a lot of referred patients from other areas of the city.

  Do you re-assign your best Rep to handle new territory?

- You assigned individual Rep's specific presentations for a District Sales Meeting. Your top performer and most experienced Rep was not prepared for his assignment and obviously put little time into preparation.

  Do you: Let it go? Bring it up immediately? Bring it up on the next working trip?

DECISION MAKING

We saved Decision Making to last because we feel confident in saying that your success, and your Representatives' success, depends on your ability to make decisions fairly, quickly and decisively. Whether it is a decision on ranking a Rep's performance or deciding what each Rep should receive as a yearly sales quota, making decisions, in our opinion, is probably the most important aspect of management. And, something that you do every day

The Urban. J. "Joe" Hecker School of Management taught us how to make decisions. Here is what Joe taught us:

Picture a square with a line in the middle running from north to south and a line in the middle of the square running from east to west so that you have 4 boxes the same size.

- In the upper left square of the box you write *"too much"*

- In the upper right square of the box you write *"too soon"*

- In the lower left square of the box you write *"too little"*

- In the lower right square of the box you write *"too late"*

- In the center of the box you draw a circle and write the words *"just right"*

Print this diagram with the four boxes and the circle in the middle and put it on your bulletin board at your desk. Every time you have a decision to make, look at where the decision you are making falls in the box.

Is the decision you are making *"too late"*

Or are you making the decision *"too soon"?*

or is it *"too early"* to make the decision?

Or is there *"too little"* information to make a decision?

Be willing to make decisions. That is the most important quality in a good leader. Avoid the *"Ready-aim-aim-aim-aim"* syndrome. You have to be willing to fire.

THE FINAL PAGE...

There are many, many good books available on leadership, and the one we like best and would encourage you, as a new or experienced manager, to read is *"Wooden On Leadership: How To Create A Winning Organization"*.

In addition, we would encourage you to read and take time to think about our "**Management Maxims**". These are rules of conduct and elements of management we would strongly encourage you to think about and apply, particularly the maxim of sharing information with your team. While many things have changed over the years, these "**Maxims**" have withstood the test of time.

Everything written in this book came from years of observation and experience in managing office-based and teaching hospital-based pharma representatives on the front-line, and our experiences managing PharmD's and PhD's calling on nationally recognized clinician thought leaders. We made mistakes as new managers, and we hope what we learned will be of value and will assist you in avoiding our mistakes.

Look for what your representatives are doing right and build on those strengths is what we learned in Urban "Joe" Hecker's School of Management. Hands down the best teacher we ever had. He taught us the importance of communication and team building. Take care and be mindful of the little things he preached. As new District Managers, ,the first thing he taught us was the importance of making decisions.

<u>A final thought</u>…Warren Buffett believes that there is one habit which separates successful people from the crowd. His quote:

"The difference between successful people and really successful people is that really successful people say 'no' to almost everything"

Keep control of your time. Say *'no'* to unimportant things coming your way on a daily basis, and stay focused on saying *'yes'* to a few things that truly matter. Set your own agenda, don't let people set your agenda for you.

We value your opinion…please send us your comments and ideas. We hope to share them with our readers.

We would encourage you to also read two other books we have written in the pharmaceutical arena.

The first book, *"**How To Sell Pharmaceuticals and Medical Devices When You Are Really Not Sure How**"* goes into how to get a provider to prescribe a drug for the very first time and includes an in-depth section on how providers are trained to think and make drug selection decisions. Further, it goes into detail explain *"patient-type centered selling"©* and how to present a product which makes the most sense to a provider.

The second book, **"*Analyzing, Interpreting & Understanding The Medical Literature*"** teaches the reader how to break down a medical study, how to spot bias and how present a study to a practitioner in 30-second and stand-up presentations. Even if your company does not allow representatives to use medical journal studies in sales presentations, this book will help you better understand your promotional marketing background and insight into the way your marketing and sales points were clinically studied.

Ron Sheeley rsheeley09@gmail.com

Paul Snyder psnyder1@indy.rr.com

Sheeleyconsulting.com

"Keep it simple, be practical and get a raise "
—Urban J Hecker, Chicago, IL, circa 1986